AIR FRYER Recipes

Unleash the Magic of Air Fryer Cooking and Indulge in Irresistible Flavors.

Lisa Johnson

© Copyright 2023 by **Lisa Johnson** - All rights reserved.

The following Book is reproduced below with the goal of providing information that is as accurate and reliable as possible. Regardless, purchasing this Book can be seen as consent to the fact that both the publisher and the author of this book are in no way experts on the topics discussed within and that any recommendations or suggestions that are made herein are for entertainment purposes only. Professionals should be consulted as needed prior to undertaking any of the action endorsed herein.

This declaration is deemed fair and valid by both the American Bar Association and the Committee of Publishers Association and is legally binding throughout the United States.

Furthermore, the transmission, duplication, or reproduction of any of the following work including specific information will be considered an illegal act irrespective of if it is done electronically or in print. This extends to creating a secondary or tertiary copy of the work or a recorded copy and is only allowed with the express written consent from the Publisher. All additional right reserved.

The information in the following pages is broadly considered a truthful and accurate account of facts and as such, any inattention, use, or misuse of the information in question by the reader will render any resulting actions solely under their purview. There are no scenarios in which the publisher or the original author of this work can be in any fashion deemed liable for any hardship or damages that may befall them after undertaking information described herein.

Additionally, the information in the following pages is intended only for informational purposes and should thus be thought of as universal. As befitting its nature, it is presented without assurance regarding its prolonged validity or interim quality. Trademarks that are mentioned are done without written consent and can in no way be considered an endorsement from the trademark holder.

All picture are under licence by CC BY-SA-NC and CC BY-NC

Table of content

American-Style Roast Beef 1

Argentinian Beef Empanadas 4

Authentic Greek Souvlaki with Sauce 7

Barbecue Skirt Steak 10

BBQ Glazed Beef Riblets 13

Beef and Broccoli Stir-Fry 16

Beef Parmigiana Sliders 19

Beef Sausage-Stuffed Zucchini 22

Beef Taco Roll-Ups with Cotija Cheese 25

Chicago-Style Beef Sandwich 28

Chuck Roast with Rustic Potatoes 31

Classic Beef Jerky 34

Crustless Beef and Cheese Tart 37

Cuban Mojo Beef 40

Dad's Barbecued Ribs 43

Dad's Meatloaf with a Twist 46

Dijon Top Chuck with Herbs 49

Doubly Cheesy Meatballs 51

Easy Beef Burritos 54

Filet Mignon and Green Bean Salad 57

Grandma's Meat Tarts 60

Grandma's Roast Beef with Harvest Vegetables 62

Greek-Style Roast Beef 65

Italian Piadina Sandwich 68

Italian-Style Steak with Cremini Mushrooms 71

London Broil with Herb Butter 73

Marinated London Broil 76

Mayo Roasted Sirloin Steak	78
Meatballs with Cranberry Sauce	80
Mediterranean Burgers with Onion Jam	82
Mediterranean-Style Beef Steak and Zucchini	84
New York Strip with Mustard Butter	86
Peperonata with Beef Sausage	88
Porterhouse Steak with Tangy Sauce	90
Roasted Ribeye with Garlic Mayo	92
Scotch Fillet with Sweet 'n' Sticky Sauce	94
Sunday Beef Schnitzel	96
Taco Stuffed Avocados	98
Tex-Mex Taco Pizza	100
Traditional Italian Beef Braciole	102
Alphabetical Index	104

American-Style Roast Beef

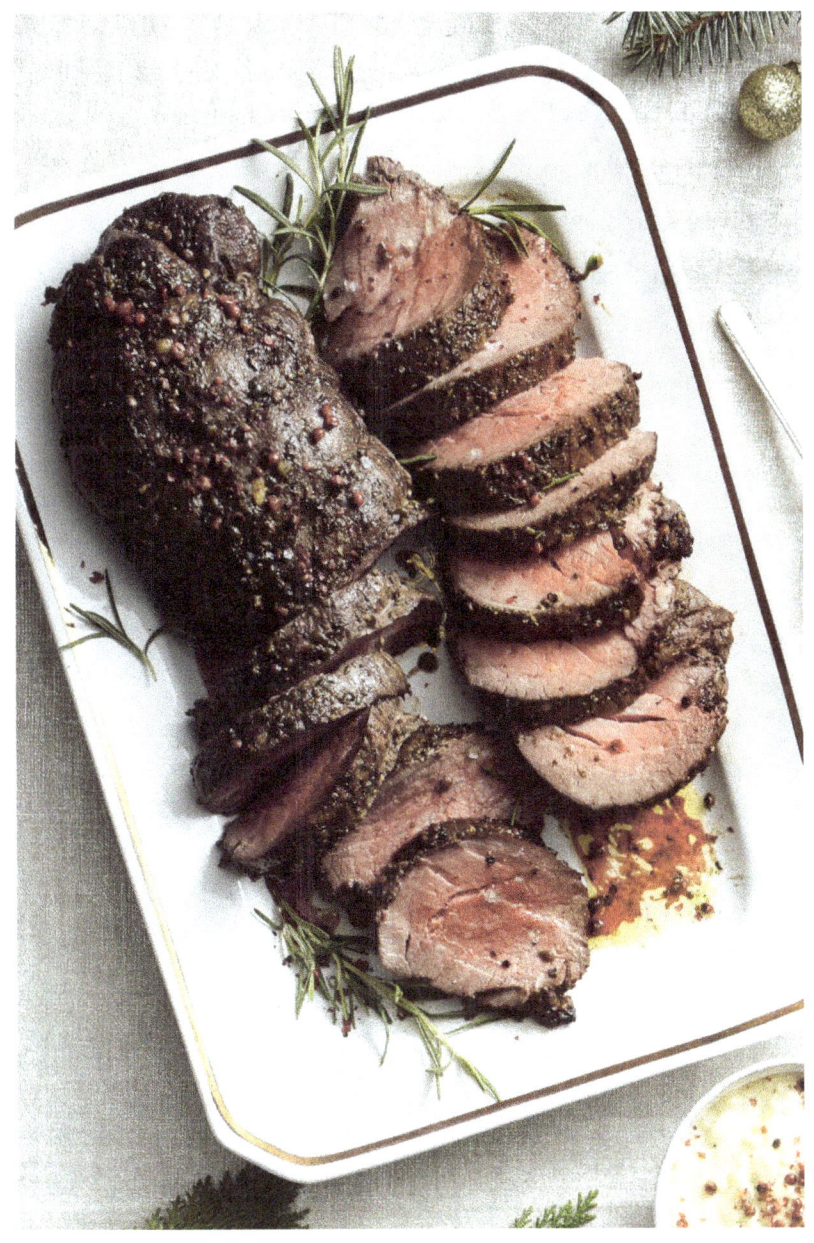

(Ready in about 30 minutes | Servings 3)

Per serving:

294 Calories; 10.9g Fat; 0.3g Carbs; 45.9g Protein; 0.3g Sugars

Ingredients

1 pound beef eye of round roast 1 teaspoon sesame oil

1 teaspoon red pepper flakes

1/4 teaspoon dried bay laurel 1/2 teaspoon cumin powder

Sea salt and black pepper, to taste

1 sprig thyme, crushed

Directions

Simply toss the beef with the remaining Ingredients; toss until well coated on all sides.

Cook in the preheated Air Fryer at 390 degrees F for 15 to 20 minutes, flipping the meat halfway through to cook on the other side.

Remove from the cooking basket, cover loosely with foil and let rest for 15 minutes before carving and serving. Bon appétit!

Argentinian Beef Empanadas

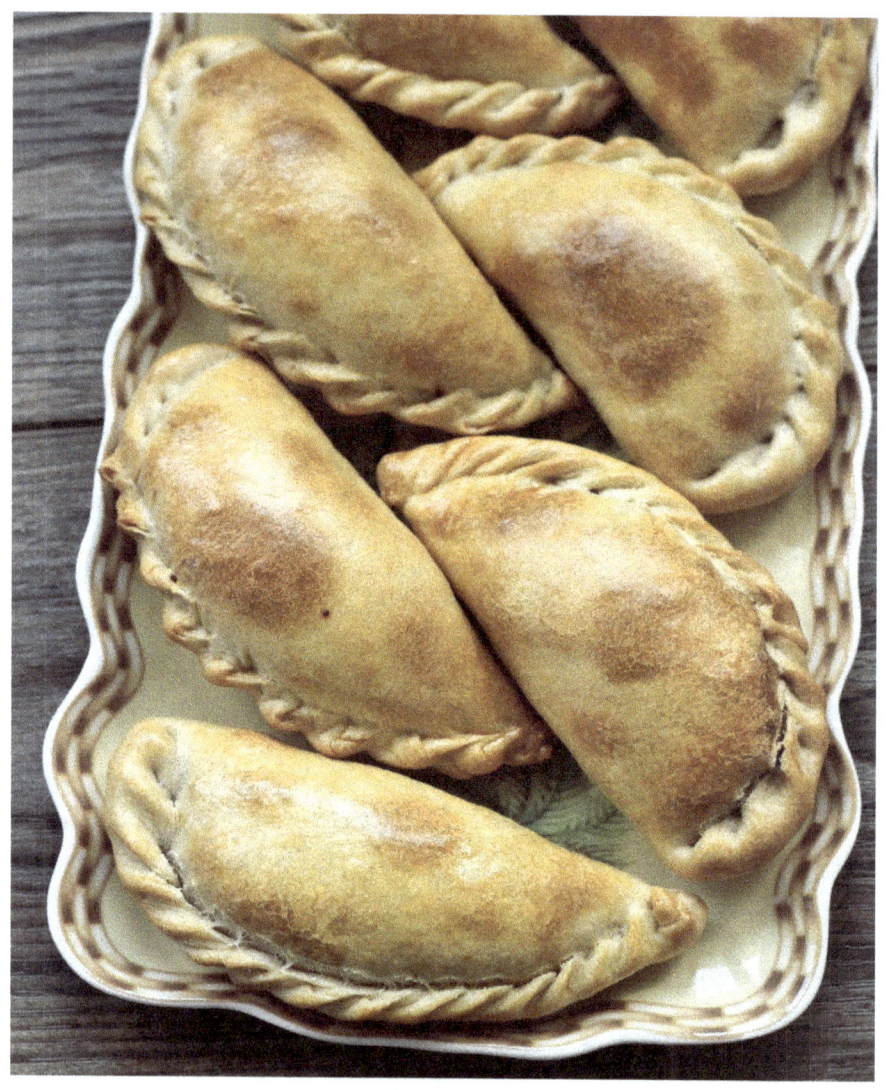

(Ready in about 20 minutes | Servings 2)

Per serving:

630 Calories; 27.3g Fat; 72g Carbs; 22g Protein; 9.7g Sugars

Ingredients

1/2 pound ground chuck 1/2 yellow onion

1 teaspoon fresh garlic, minced

2 tablespoons piri piri sauce 1 tablespoon mustard

6 cubes Cotija cheese

6 Goya discos pastry dough

Directions

Heat a nonstick skillet over medium-high heat. Once hot, cook the ground beef, onion and garlic until tender, about 6 minutes. Crumble with a fork and stir in the piri piri sauce; stir to combine.

Divide the sauce between empanadas. Top with mustard and cheese. Fold each of them in half and seal the edges.

Bake in the preheated Air Fryer at 340 degrees F for about 8 minutes, flipping them halfway through the cooking time. Serve with salsa sauce if desired.

Authentic Greek Souvlaki with Sauce

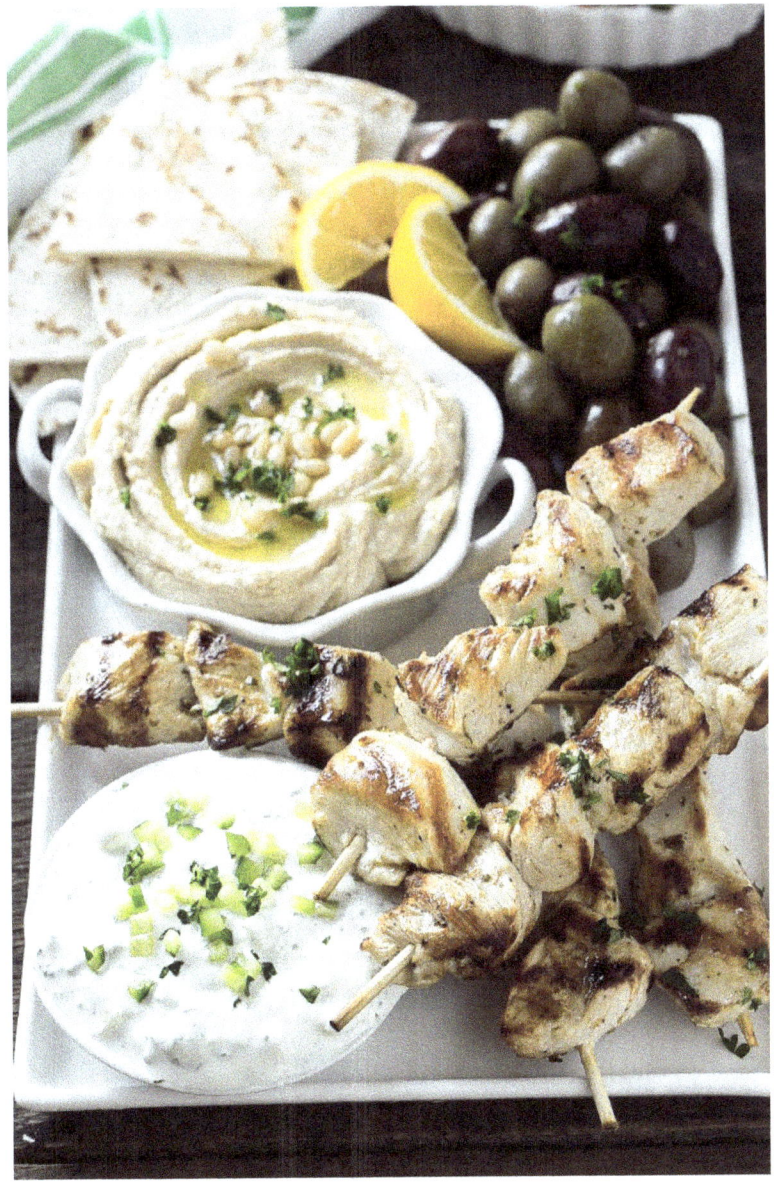

(Ready in about 15 minutes + marinating time | Servings 2)0

Per serving:

366 Calories; 20.7g Fat; 14.8g Carbs; 26.3g Protein; 10.1g Sugars

Ingredients

1/2 pound sirloin steak, cut into bite-sized pieces 1 tablespoon olive oil

2 tablespoons Worcestershire sauce 4 tablespoons wine vinegar

1 tablespoon molasses

1 tablespoon mustard

2 garlic cloves, pressed

1 teaspoon dried oregano 1/4 teaspoon sea salt

1 teaspoon black peppercorns

4 tablespoons Greek-style yogurt 1/2 teaspoon tzatziki spice mix

2 tablespoons mayonnaise

4 wooden skewer sticks, soaked in water

Directions

Place the sirloin steak, olive oil, Worcestershire sauce, vinegar, molasses, mustard, garlic, oregano, salt and black peppercorns in a ceramic dish.

Place in your refrigerator and let it marinate overnight.

Thread the beef cubes onto skewers. Cook in preheated Air Fryer at 395 degrees F for 12 minutes, flipping halfway through the cooking time.

In the meantime, mix the Greek yogurt with the tzatziki spice mix and mayo. Serve the souvlaki with the sauce on the side.

Barbecue Skirt Steak

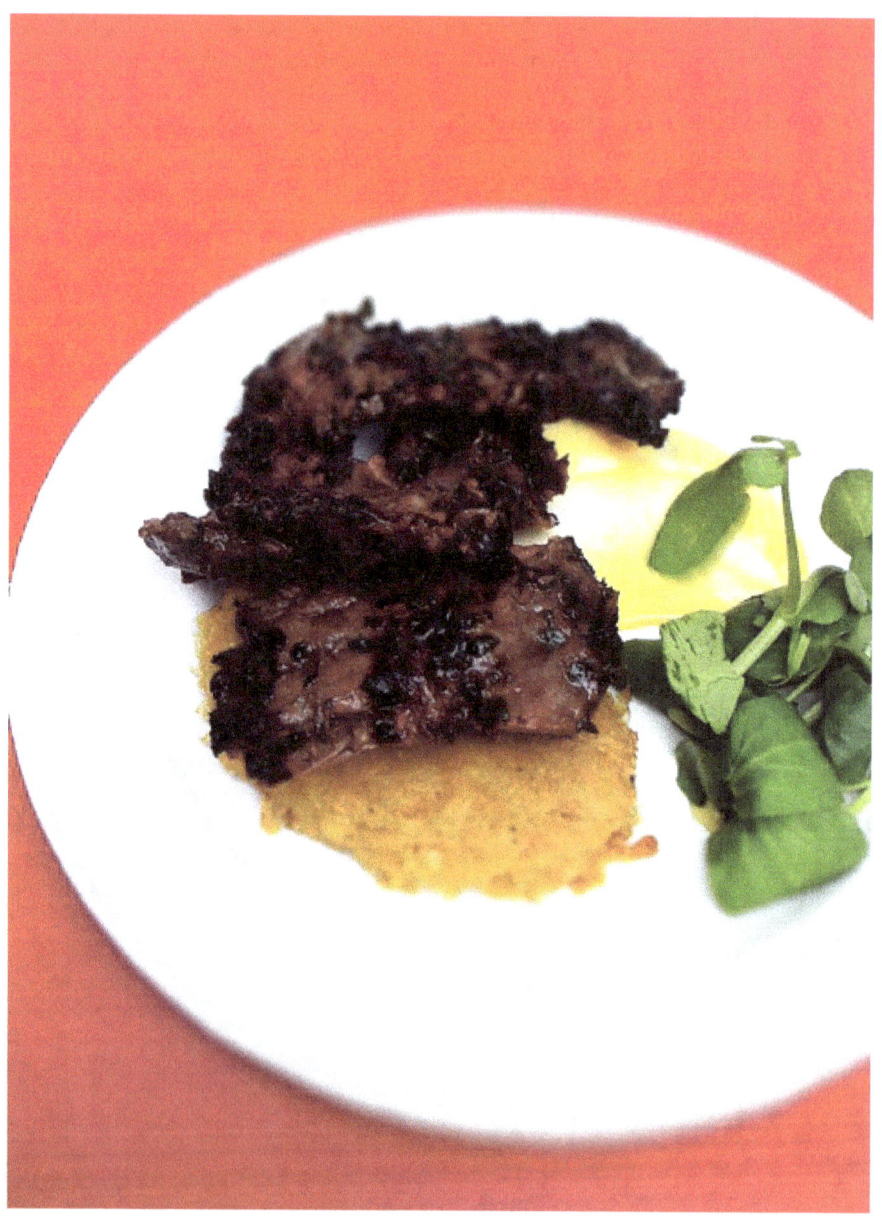

(Ready in about 20 minutes + marinating time | Servings 5)

Per serving:

394 Calories; 19g Fat; 4.4g Carbs; 51.3g Protein; 3.3g Sugars

Ingredients

2 pounds skirt steak

2 tablespoons tomato paste 1 tablespoon tomato ketchup 1 tablespoon olive oil

1 tablespoon soy sauce 1/4 cup rice vinegar

1 tablespoon fish sauce Sea salt, to taste

1/2 teaspoon dried dill

1/2 teaspoon dried rosemary

1/4 teaspoon black pepper, freshly cracked 1 tablespoon brown sugar

Directions

Place all Ingredients in a large ceramic dish; let it marinate for 3 hours in your refrigerator.

Coat the sides and bottom of the Air Fryer with cooking spray.

Add your steak to the cooking basket; reserve the marinade. Cook the skirt steak in the preheated Air Fryer at 400 degrees F for 12 minutes, turning over a couple of times, basting with the reserved marinade.

Serve warm with roasted new potatoes, if desired.

BBQ Glazed Beef Riblets

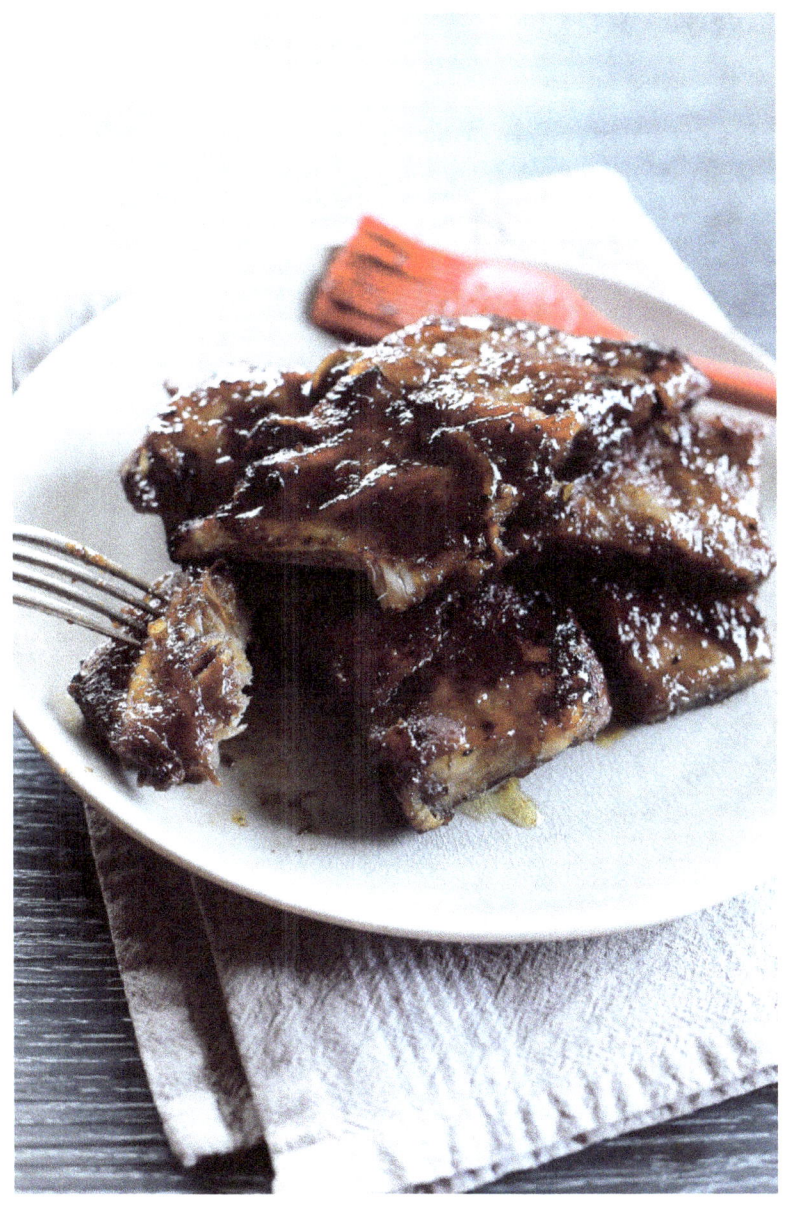

(Ready in about 15 minutes + marinating time | Servings 3)

Per serving:

258 Calories; 9.5g Fat; 10.4g Carbs; 32.7g Protein; 5.3g Sugars

Ingredients

1 pound beef riblets

Sea salt and red pepper, to taste 1/4 cup tomato paste

1/4 cup Worcestershire sauce 2 tablespoons hot sauce

1 tablespoon oyster sauce

2 tablespoons rice vinegar

1 tablespoon stone-ground mustard

Directions

Combine all Ingredients in a glass dish, cover and marinate at least 2 hours in your refrigerator.

Discard the marinade and place riblets in the Air Fryer cooking basket.

Cook in the preheated Air Fryer at 360 degrees F for 12 minutes, shaking the basket halfway through to ensure even cooking.

Heat the reserved marinade in a small skillet over a moderate flame; spoon the glaze over the riblets and serve immediately.

Beef and Broccoli Stir-Fry

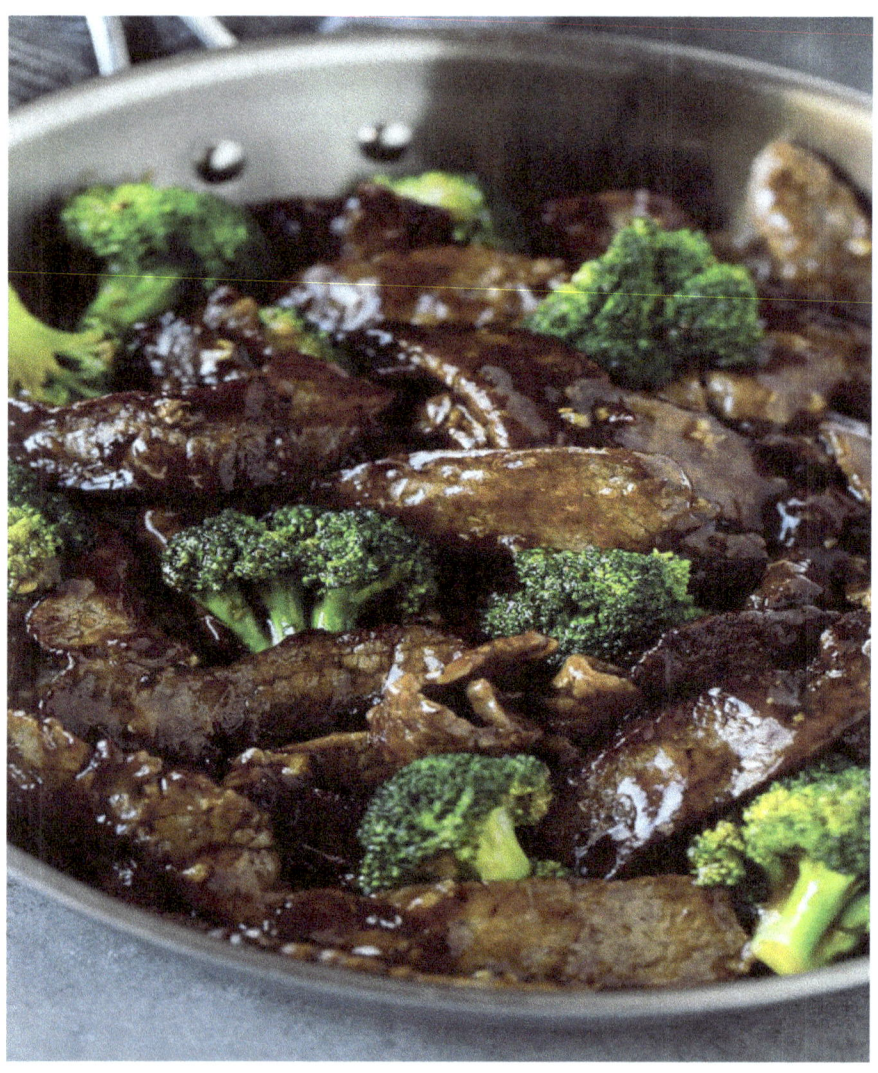

(Ready in about 20 minutes | Servings 2)

Per serving:

500 Calories; 23.1g Fat; 9.2g Carbs; 65g Protein; 2.4g Sugars

Ingredients

1/2 pound beef stew meat, cut into bite-sized cubes 1/2 pound broccoli, cut into florets

1 small shallot, sliced

1 teaspoon peanut oil

1/2 teaspoon garlic powder Salt and red pepper, to taste

1 teaspoon Five-spice powder 1 tablespoon fish sauce

1 tablespoon tamari sauce

1 teaspoon sesame seed oil

1 teaspoon Chiu Chow chili sauce

Directions

Toss all Ingredients until the beef and veggies are well coated.

Cook in the preheated Air Fryer at 400 degrees F for 6 minutes; shake the basket and continue to air fry for 6 minutes more.

Now, test the meat for doneness, remove the vegetables and cook the meat for 5 minutes more if needed.

Taste and adjust seasonings. Serve immediately.

Beef Parmigiana Sliders

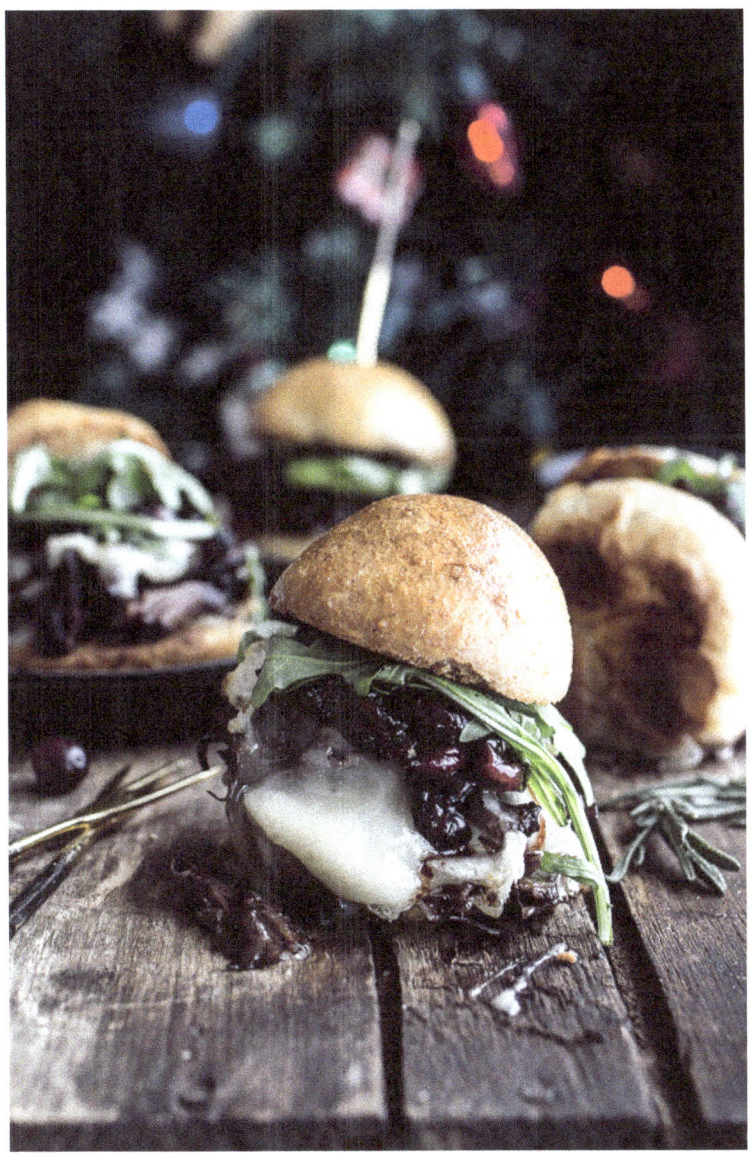

(Ready in about 15 minutes | Servings 2)

Per serving:

516 Calories; 20.7g Fat; 42g Carbs; 34.3g Protein; 5.1g Sugars

Ingredients

1/2 pound lean ground chuck 1 ounce bacon bits

2 tablespoons tomato paste

3 tablespoons shallots, chopped 1 garlic clove, minced

1/4 cup parmesan cheese, grated

1 teaspoon cayenne pepper Salt and black pepper, to taste 4 pretzel rolls

Directions

Thoroughly combine the ground chuck, bacon bits, tomato paste, shallots, garlic, parmesan cheese, cayenne pepper, salt, black pepper.

Shape the mixture into 4 equal patties.

Spritz your patties with a nonstick cooking spray. Air fry your burgers at 380 degrees F for about 11 minutes or to your desired degree of doneness.

Place your burgers on pretzel rolls and serve with favorite toppings. Enjoy!

Beef Sausage-Stuffed Zucchini

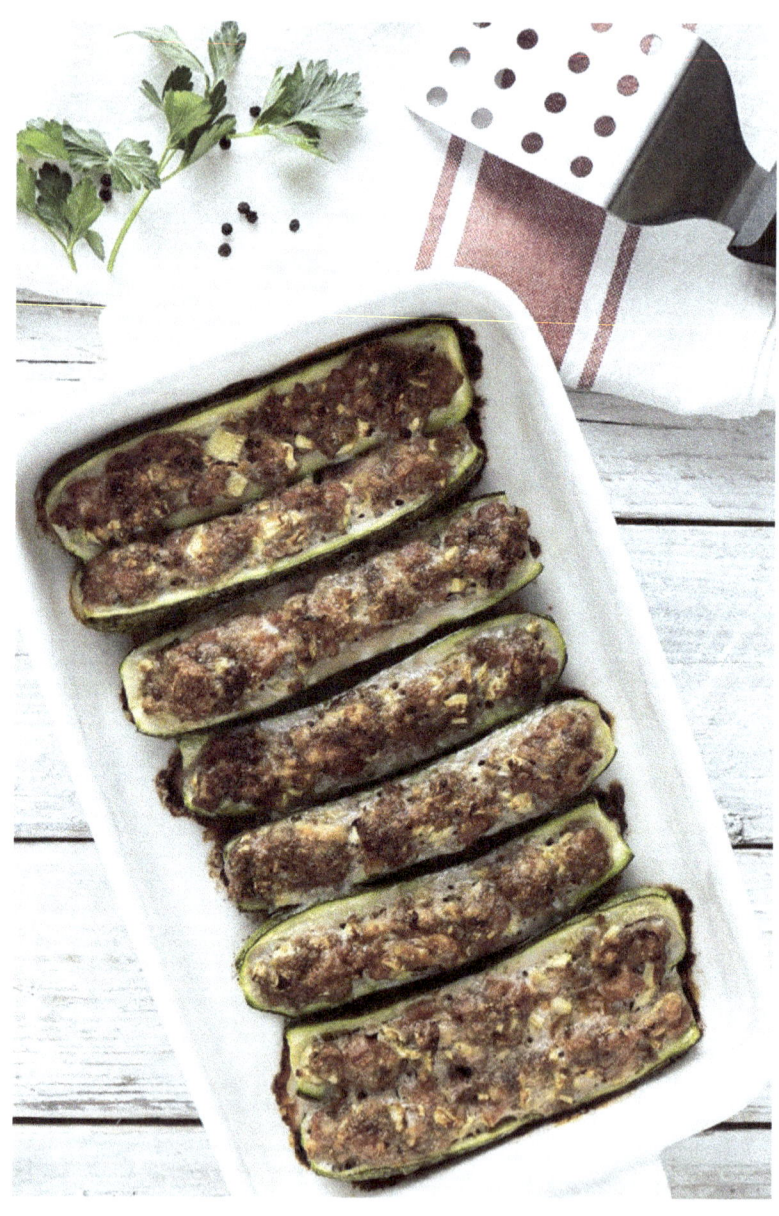

(Ready in about 30 minutes | Servings 2)

Per serving:

435 Calories; 28g Fat; 19.3g Carbs; 26.5g Protein; 7.7g Sugars

Ingredients

1/2 pound beef sausage, crumbled 1/2 cup tortilla chips, crushed

1/2 teaspoon garlic, pressed

1/4 cup tomato paste

2 small-sized zucchini, halved lengthwise and seeds removed 1/2 cup sharp cheddar cheese, grated

Directions

In a mixing bowl, thoroughly combine the beef sausage, tortilla chips, garlic and tomato paste. Divide the sausage mixture between the zucchini halves.

Bake in the preheated Air Fryer at 400 degrees F for 20 minutes.

Top with grated cheddar cheese and cook an additional 5 minutes. Enjoy!

Beef Taco Roll-Ups with Cotija Cheese

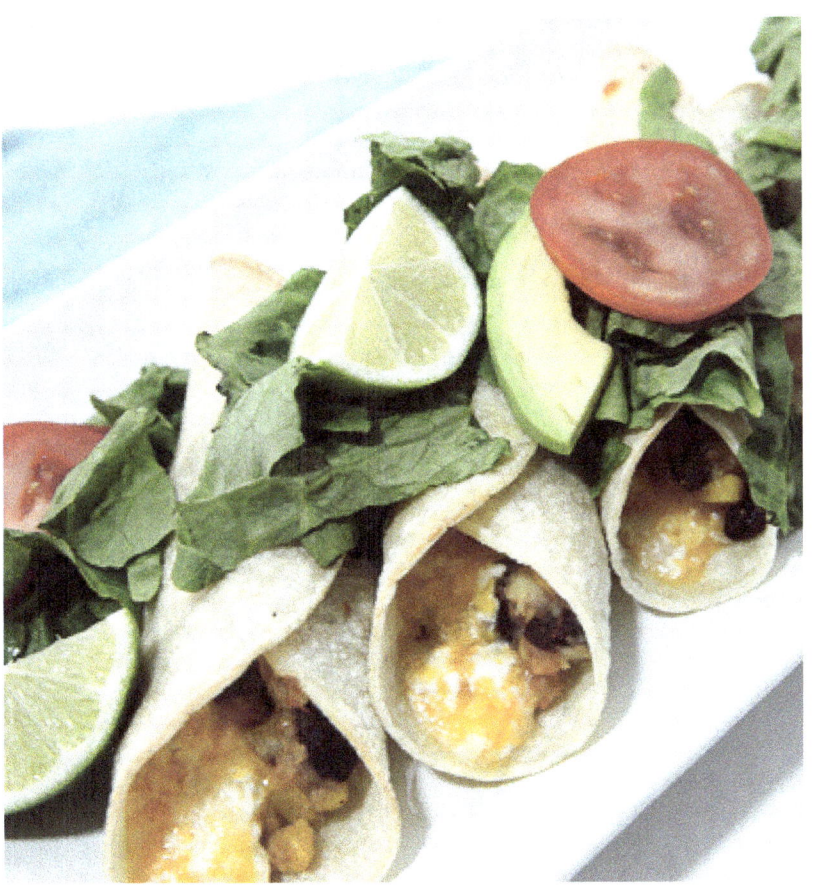

(Ready in about 25 minutes | Servings 4)

Per serving:

417 Calories; 15.9g Fat; 41g Carbs; 26.2g Protein; 1.5g Sugars

Ingredients

1 tablespoon sesame oil

2 tablespoons scallions, chopped 1 garlic clove, minced

1 bell pepper, chopped 1/2 pound ground beef

1/2 teaspoon Mexican oregano

1/2 teaspoon dried marjoram 1 teaspoon chili powder

1/2 cup refried beans

Sea salt and ground black pepper, to taste 1/2 cup Cotija cheese, shredded

8 roll wrappers

Directions

Start by preheating your Air Fryer to 395 degrees F.

Heat the sesame oil in a nonstick skillet over medium-high heat. Cook the scallions, garlic, and peppers until tender and fragrant.

Add the ground beef, oregano, marjoram, and chili powder. Continue cooking for 3 minutes longer or until it is browned.

Stir in the beans, salt, and pepper. Divide the meat/bean mixture between wrappers that are softened with a little bit of water. Top with cheese.

Roll the wrappers and spritz them with cooking oil on all sides.

Cook in the preheated Air Fryer for 11 to 12 minutes, flipping them halfway through the cooking time. Enjoy!

Chicago-Style Beef Sandwich

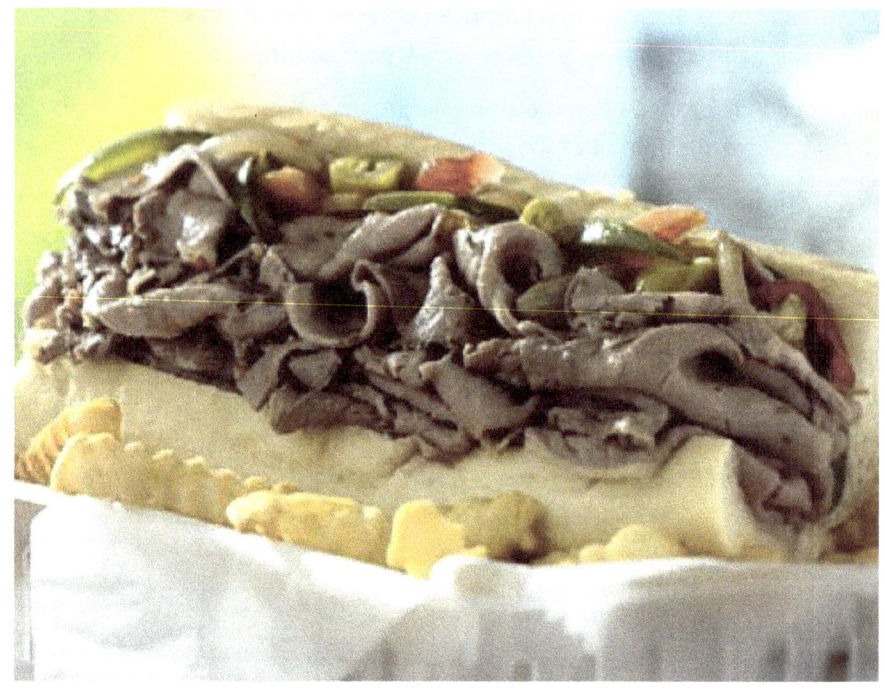

(Ready in about 25 minutes | Servings 2)

Per serving:

385 Calories; 17.4g Fat; 28.1g Carbs; 29.8g Protein; 6.2g Sugars

Ingredients

1/2 pound chuck, boneless 1 tablespoon olive oil

1 tablespoon soy sauce

1/4 teaspoon ground bay laurel 1/2 teaspoon shallot powder 1/4 teaspoon porcini powder 1/2 teaspoon garlic powder

1/2 teaspoon cayenne pepper

Kosher salt and ground black pepper, to taste 1 cup pickled vegetables, chopped

2 ciabatta rolls, sliced in half

Directions

Toss the chuck roast with olive oil, soy sauce and spices until well coated.

Cook in the preheated Air Fryer at 400 degrees F for 20 minutes, turning over halfway through the cooking time.

Shred the meat with two forks and adjust seasonings.

Top the bottom halves of the ciabatta rolls with a generous portion of the meat and pickled vegetables. Place the tops of the ciabatta rolls on the sandwiches. Serve immediately and enjoy!

Chuck Roast with Rustic Potatoes

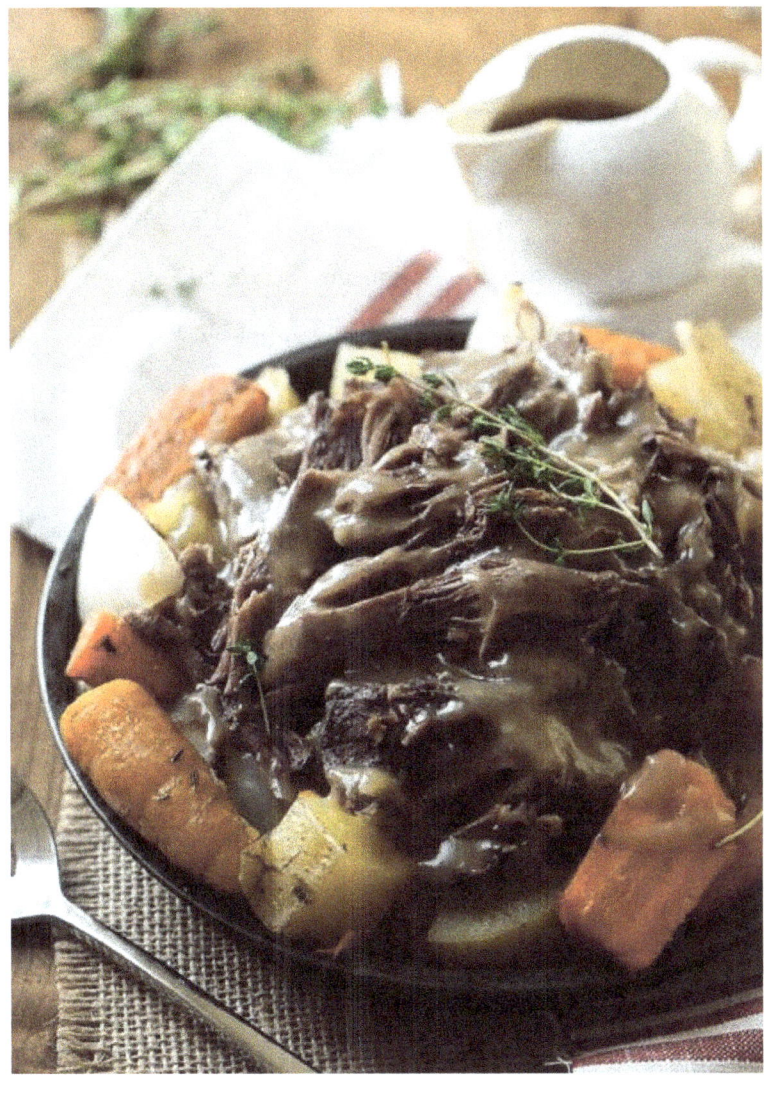

(Ready in about 50 minutes | Servings 3)

Per serving:

438 Calories; 13.1g Fat; 30.8g Carbs; 50g Protein; 2.9g Sugars

Ingredients

1 tablespoon brown mustard

2 tablespoons tomato paste, preferably homemade

2 tablespoons BBQ sauce

1 tablespoon Worcester sauce 1 ½ pounds chuck roast

1 pound medium-sized russet potatoes, quartered

Coarse sea salt and ground black pepper, to taste 1/2 teaspoon cayenne pepper

1 teaspoon shallot powder

1 teaspoon granulated garlic 1 teaspoon dried marjoram

Directions

Mix the mustard, tomato paste, BBQ sauce and Worcester sauce in a small bowl. Rub this mixture all over the chuck roast.

Add spices and place the chuck roast in the Air Fryer cooking basket that is lightly greased with melted butter.

Air fry at 400 degrees F for 30 minutes; turn it over and scatter potato chunks around the beef. Continue to cook an additional 15 minutes. Double check to make sure the beef is cooked thoroughly.

Taste and adjust seasonings. Place the meat on a cutting board. Slice the beef against the grain and eat warm.

Classic Beef Jerky

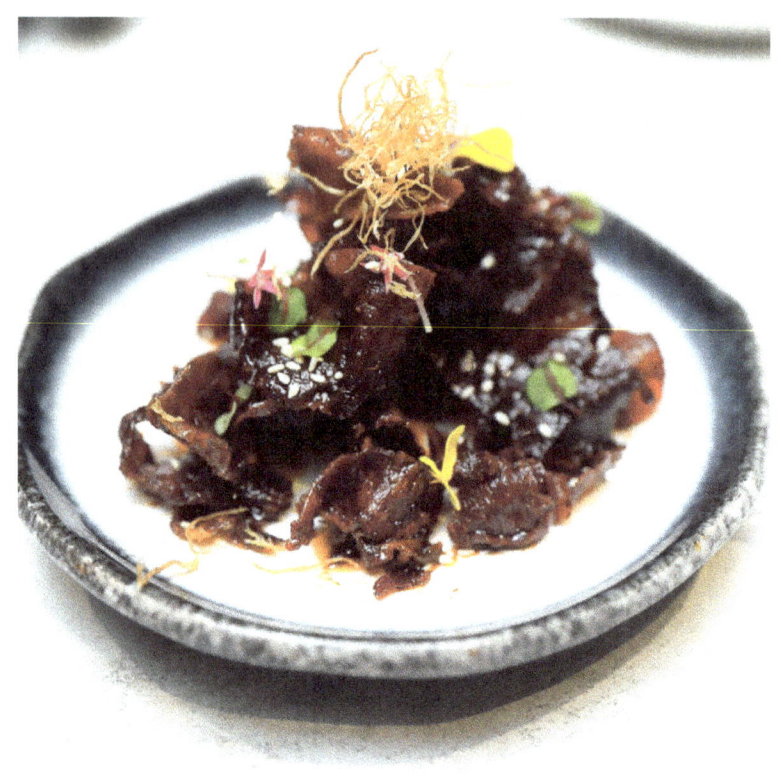

(Ready in about 4 hours 30 minutes | Servings 4)

Per serving:

77 Calories; 2.4g Fat; 4.1g Carbs; 8.9g Protein; 3.1g Sugars

Ingredients

6 ounces top round steak, cut into 1/8-inch thick strips 1/2 teaspoon fresh garlic, crushed

1 teaspoon onion powder

2 tablespoons Worcestershire sauce 1/2 tablespoon honey

1 teaspoon liquid smoke

1 teaspoon hot sauce

Directions

Transfer the strips of steak to a large Ziplock bag; add in the other Ingredients, seal the bag and shake to combine well.

Refrigerate for at least 30 minutes.

Cook in the preheated Air Fryer at 160 degrees F for about 4 hours, until it is dry and firm.

Refrigerate in an airtight container for up to 1 month. Bon appétit!

Crustless Beef and Cheese Tart

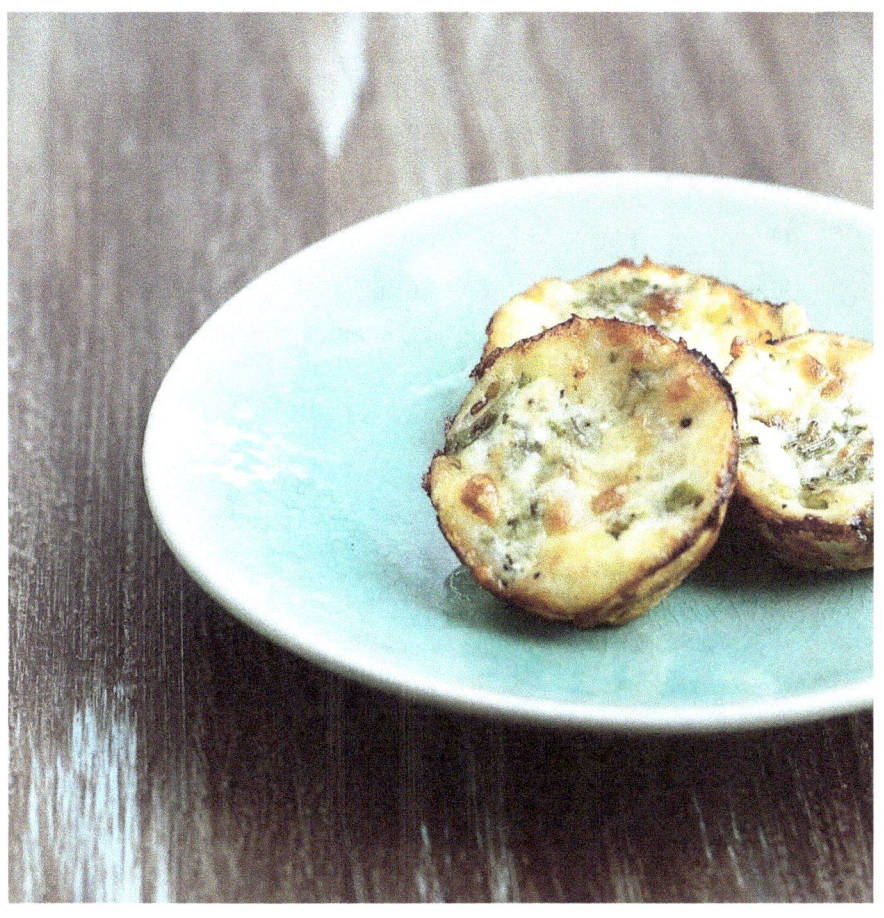

(Ready in about 25 minutes | Servings 4)

Per serving:

572 Calories; 44.6g Fat; 16.2g Carbs; 28.1g Protein; 8.9g Sugars

Ingredients

1 tablespoon canola oil 1 onion, finely chopped

2 fresh garlic cloves, minced

1/2 pound ground chuck

1/2 pound Chorizo sausage, crumbled 1 cup pasta sauce

Sea salt, to taste

1/4 teaspoon ground black pepper

1/2 teaspoon red pepper flakes, crushed 1 cup cream cheese, room temperature 1/2 cup Swiss cheese, shredded

1 egg

1/2 cup crackers, crushed

Directions

Start by preheating your Air Fryer to 370 degrees F. Grease a baking pan with canola oil.

Add the onion, garlic, ground chuck, sausage, pasta sauce, salt, black pepper, and red pepper. Cook for 9 minutes.

In the meantime, combine cheese with egg. Place the cheese-egg mixture over the beef mixture.

Sprinkle with crushed crackers and cook for 10 minutes. Serve warm and enjoy!

Cuban Mojo Beef

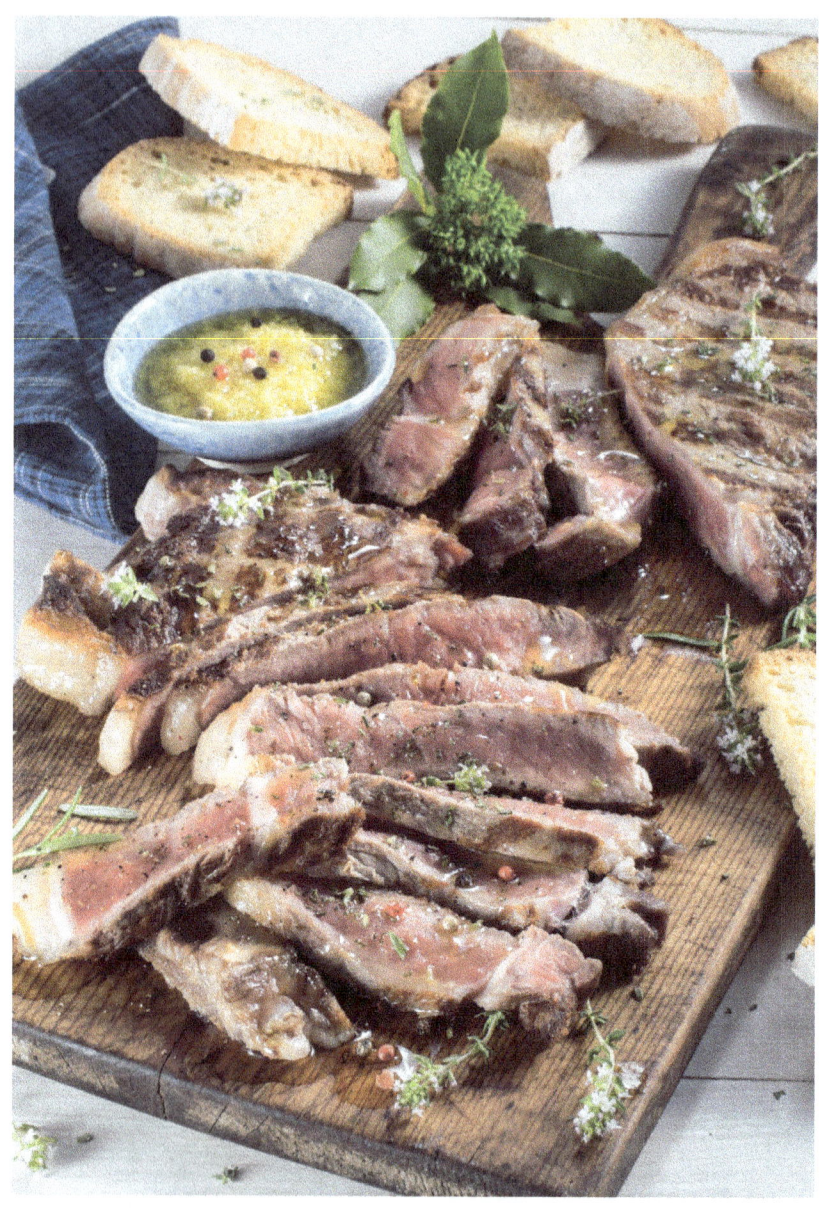

(Ready in about 15 minutes | Servings 3)

Per serving:

263 Calories; 17.4g Fat; 4.1g Carbs; 23.5g Protein; 2g Sugars

Ingredients

3/4 pound blade steak, cut into cubes 1 teaspoon olive oil

Salt and red pepper flakes, to season

Mojo sauce:

1 teaspoon garlic, smashed

2 tablespoons extra-virgin olive oil

2 tablespoons fresh parsley, chopped 2 tablespoons fresh cilantro, chopped 1/2 lime, freshly squeezed

1 green chili pepper, minced

Directions

Toss the steak with olive oil, salt and red pepper.

Cook in your Air Fryer at 400 degrees F for 12 minutes, turning them over halfway through the cooking time.

Meanwhile, make the sauce by mixing all Ingredients in your food processor or blender. Serve the warm blade steak with the Mojo sauce on the side.

Enjoy!

Dad's Barbecued Ribs

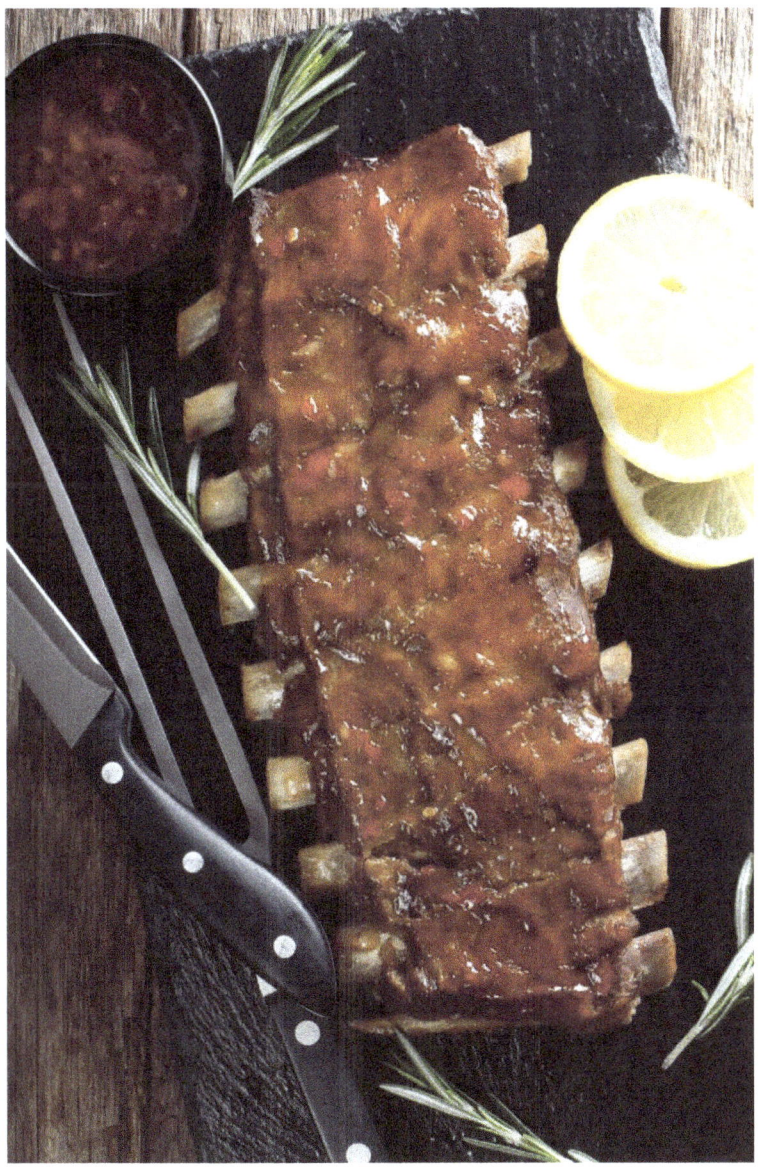

(Ready in about 20 minutes + marinating time | Servings 3)

Per serving:

566 Calories; 45g Fat; 18g Carbs; 25.7g Protein; 10.3g Sugars

Ingredients

1 pound beef ribs 1/4 cup ketchup 1/4 cup tequila

1 tablespoon brown mustard 1 tablespoon brown sugar

2 tablespoons soy sauce

1/2 red onion, sliced

2 garlic cloves, pressed

Directions

Cut the ribs into serving size portions and transfer them to a ceramic dish. Add in the remaining Ingredients, cover and allow it to marinate in your refrigerator overnight.

Discard the marinade. Grill in the preheated Air Fryer at 400 degrees F for 10 minutes. Turn them over and continue to cook for 10 minutes more.

Meanwhile, make the sauce by warming the marinade Ingredients in a nonstick pan. Spoon over the warm ribs and serve immediately.

Dad's Meatloaf with a Twist

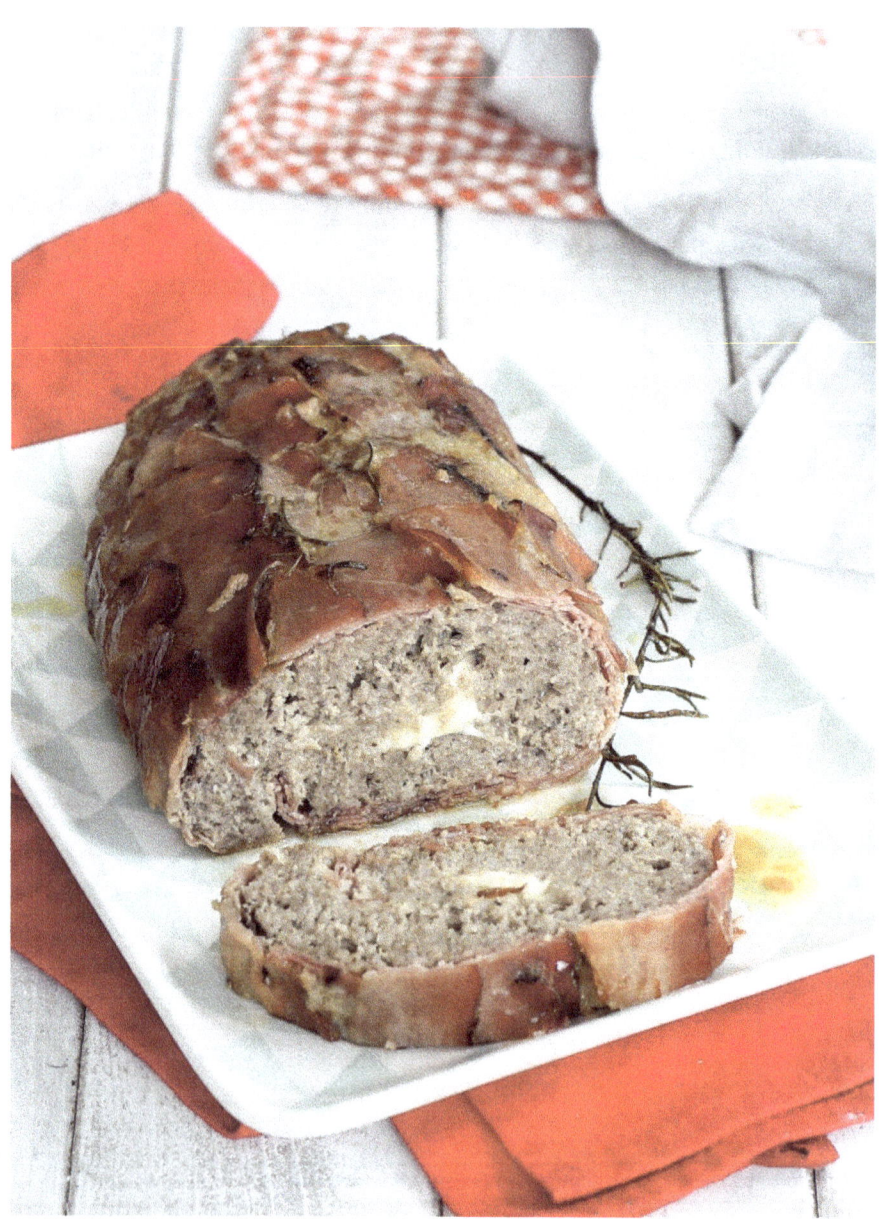

(Ready in about 35 minutes | Servings 2)

Per serving:

521 Calories; 25.5g Fat; 42.9g Carbs; 32g Protein; 9.2g Sugars

Ingredients

1 tablespoon olive oil 1 onion, chopped

1/2 teaspoon garlic, minced

1 Italian pepper, deveined and chopped 1 Serrano pepper, deveined and chopped 1/2 pound ground beef

1 tablespoon soy sauce

1 tablespoon Dijon mustard 1/2 cup crushed corn flakes 4 tablespoons tomato paste

1 teaspoon Italian seasoning mix 1/2 teaspoon liquid smoke

Directions

Start by preheating your Air Fryer to 350 degrees F.

In a mixing bowl, thoroughly combine the onion, garlic, peppers, ground beef, soy sauce, mustard and crushed corn flakes. Salt to taste.

Mix until everything is well incorporated and press into a lightly greased meatloaf pan.

Air fry for about 25 minutes. Whisk the tomato paste with the Italian seasoning mix and liquid smoke; spread the mixture over the top of your meatloaf.

Continue to cook for 3 minutes more. Let it rest for 6 minutes before slicing and serving. Bon appétit!

Dijon Top Chuck with Herbs

(Ready in about 1 hour | Servings 3)

Per serving:

406 Calories; 24.1g Fat; 0.3g Carbs; 44.1g Protein; 0g Sugars

Ingredients

1 ½ pounds top chuck 2 teaspoons olive oil

1 tablespoon Dijon mustard

Sea salt and ground black pepper, to taste 1 teaspoon dried marjoram

1 teaspoon dried thyme

1/2 teaspoon fennel seeds

Directions

Start by preheating your Air Fryer to 380 degrees F

Add all Ingredients in a Ziploc bag; shake to mix well. Next, spritz the bottom of the Air Fryer basket with cooking spray.

Place the beef in the cooking basket and cook for 50 minutes, turning every 10 to 15 minutes.

Let it rest for 5 to 7 minutes before slicing and serving. Enjoy!

Doubly Cheesy Meatballs

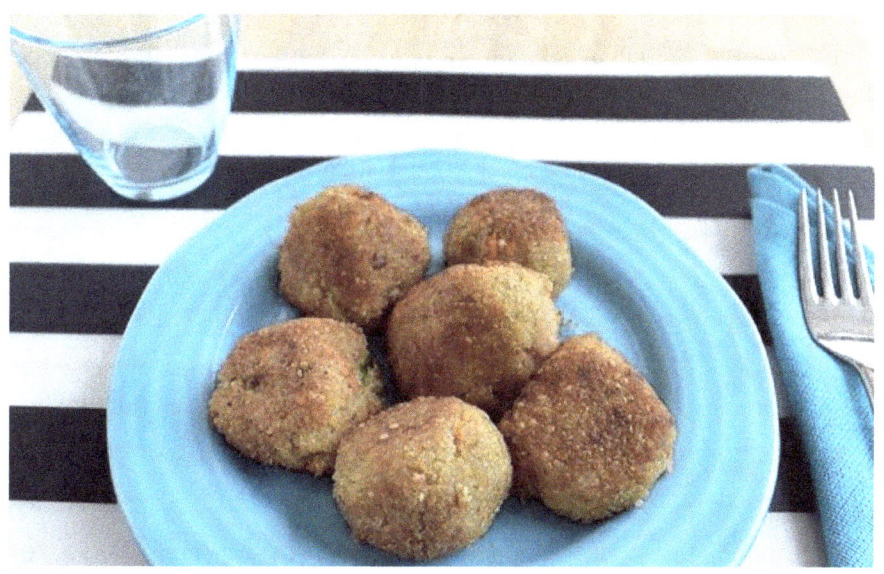

(Ready in about 15 minutes | Servings 4)

Per serving:

613 Calories; 35.1g Fat; 16.1g Carbs; 57g Protein; 2g Sugars

Ingredients

1 pound ground beef

1/4 cup Grana Padano, grated

2 tablespoons scallion, chopped 2 garlic cloves, minced

2 stale crustless bread slices

1 tablespoon Italian seasoning mix 1 egg, beaten

1/4 cup Mozzarella cheese, shredded

Kosher salt and ground black pepper, to taste

Directions

In a mixing bowl, combine all Ingredients. Then, shape the mixture into 8 meatballs.

Cook the meatballs at 370 degrees F for 10 minutes, shaking the basket halfway through the cooking time.

Serve the meatballs in a sandwich if desired.

Easy Beef Burritos

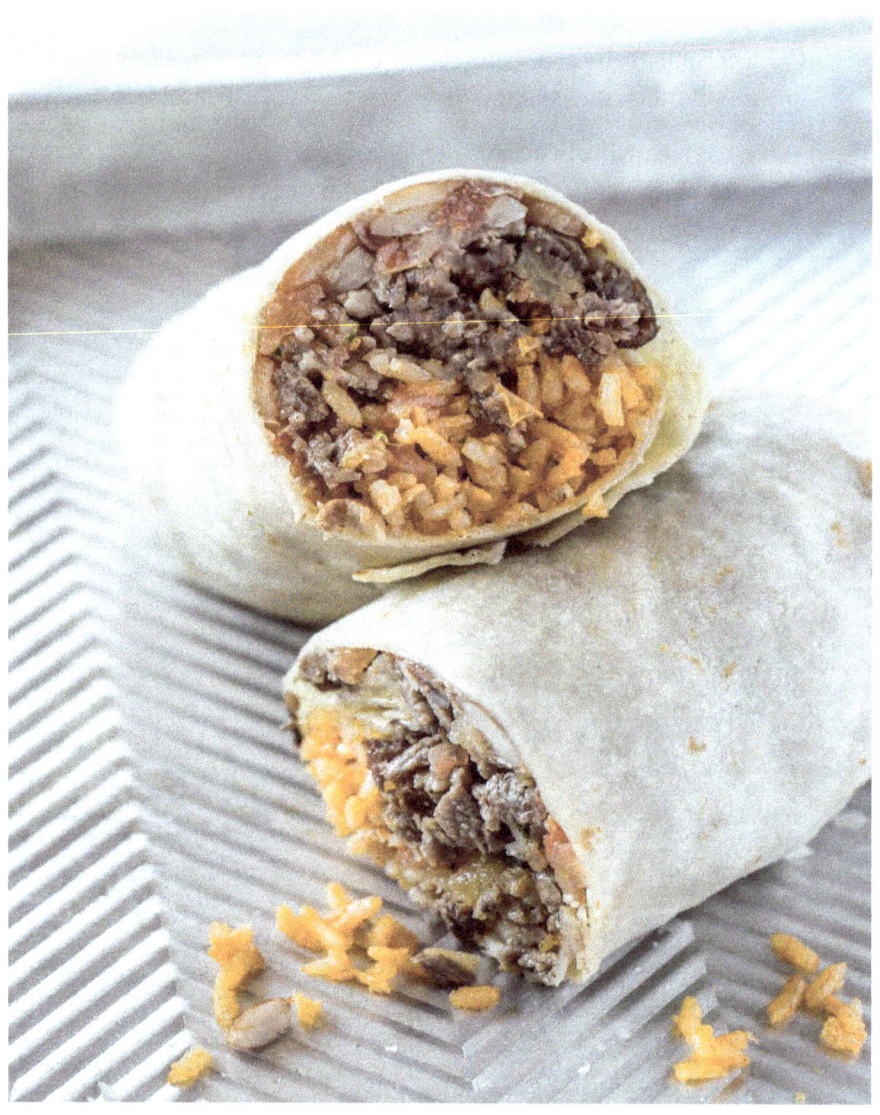

(Ready in about 25 minutes | Servings 3)

Per serving:

368 Calories; 13g Fat; 20.2g Carbs; 35.1g Protein; 2.7g Sugars

Ingredients

1 pound rump steak

Sea salt and crushed red pepper, to taste 1/2 teaspoon shallot powder

1/2 teaspoon porcini powder 1/2 teaspoon celery seeds

1/2 teaspoon dried Mexican oregano

1 teaspoon piri piri powder 1 teaspoon lard, melted

3 (approx 7-8" dia) whole-wheat tortillas

Directions

Toss the rump steak with the spices and melted lard.

Cook in your Air Fryer at 390 degrees F for 20 minutes, turning it halfway through the cooking time. Place on a cutting board to cool slightly.

Slice against the grain into thin strips.

Spoon the beef strips onto wheat tortillas; top with your favorite fixings, roll them up and serve. Enjoy!

Filet Mignon and Green Bean Salad

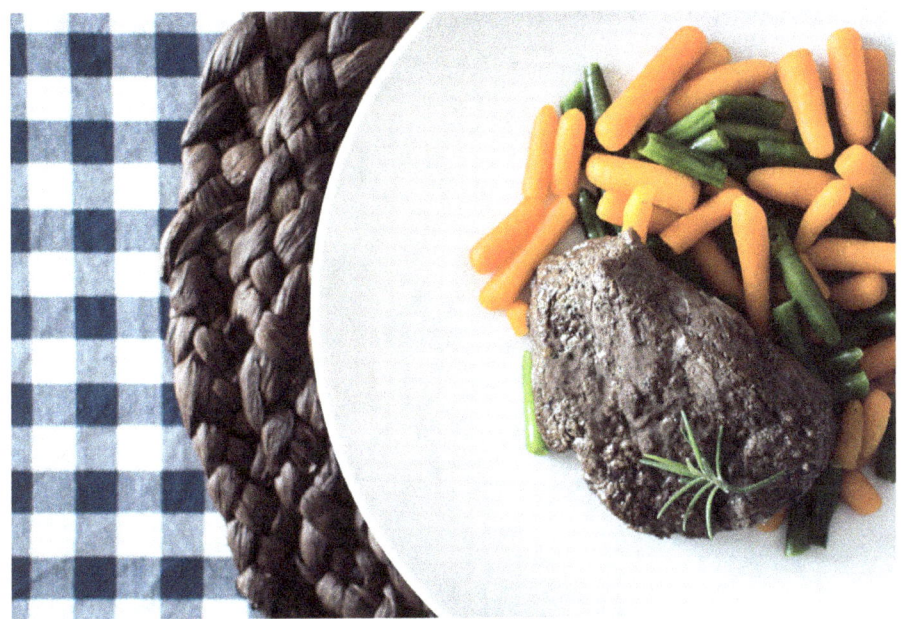

(Ready in about 25 minutes | Servings 2)

Per serving:

500 Calories; 33g Fat; 20.1g Carbs; 33.5g Protein; 8.2g Sugars

Ingredients

1/2 pound filet mignon

Salt and ground black pepper, to taste 1/2 pound green beans

1/2 teaspoon butter, melted 1 red bell pepper, sliced

1 green bell pepper, sliced

1 cup mixed greens

10 small carrots

1/4 cup walnuts, roughly chopped 1/4 cup feta cheese, crumbled

2 tablespoons tahini

1 tablespoon Dijon mustard 1 tablespoon sesame oil

1 tablespoon balsamic vinegar

2 tablespoons pomegranate seeds

Directions

Season the fillet mignon with salt and pepper to taste. Cook in the preheated Air Fryer at 400 degrees F for 18 minutes, turning them over halfway through the cooking time. Set aside.

Then, add the green beans and small carrots to the cooking basket and drizzle it with melted butter. Cook at 400 degrees F for 5 minutes, shaking the basket once or twice.

Slice the beef into bite-sized strips and transfer to a nice salad bowl.

Toss the beef and green beans with bell peppers, mixed greens, walnuts and feta cheese.

Then, make the dressing by whisking tahini, mustard, sesame oil and balsamic vinegar; dress your salad and serve garnished with pomegranate seeds. Bon appétit!

Grandma's Meat Tarts

(Ready in about 20 minutes | Servings 3)

Per serving:

496 Calories; 23.3g Fat; 41.2g Carbs; 32.3g Protein; 7g Sugars

Ingredients

6 ounces refrigerated pie crusts 3/4 pound lean ground beef 1/2 onion

1 clove garlic, finely chopped

Sea salt and ground black pepper, to taste 1/2 cup tomato paste

3 Swiss cheese slices 1 egg white, beaten

Directions

Start by preheating your Air Fryer to 360 degrees F.

Cook the ground beef, onion and garlic in a nonstick skillet until the beef is no longer pink and the onion is translucent. Season with salt and pepper; fold in the tomato paste and stir to combine.

Unroll the pie crust and use a round cookie cutter to make 3 even rounds.

Fill the pie crust rounds with the beef mixture. Top with cheese. Moisten the outside of each round with beaten egg white.

Fold the pie crust rounds in half and use a fork to gently press the edges. Cook at 360 degrees F for about 15 minutes. Serve immediately.

Grandma's Roast Beef with Harvest Vegetables

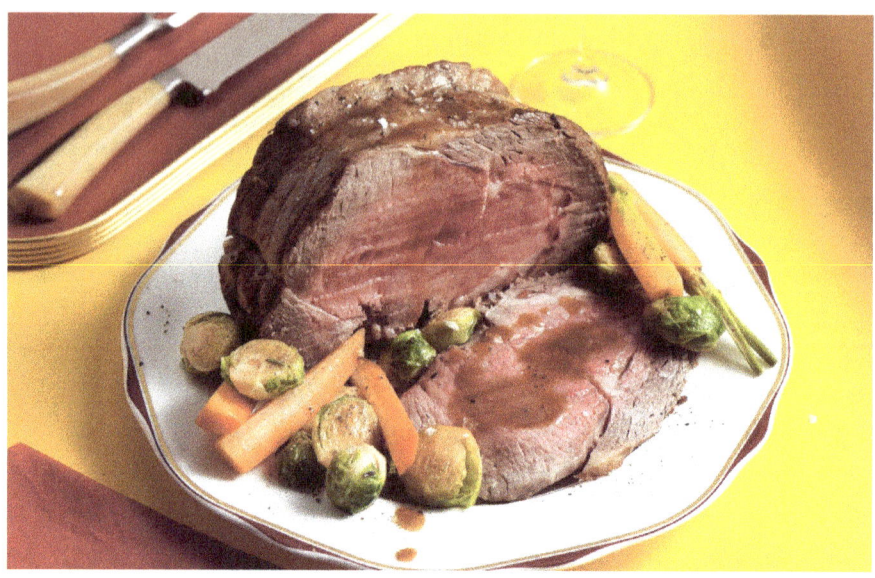

(Ready in about 45 minutes + marinating time | Servings 3)

Per serving:

272 Calories; 8.9g Fat; 17.1g Carbs; 32.1g Protein; 10.3g Sugars

Ingredients

1 pound beef roast

1 teaspoon brown mustard 1/4 cup apple juice

1 tablespoon fish sauce 1 tablespoon honey 1/2 teaspoon dried dill

1/2 teaspoon dried thyme

2 medium-sized carrots, sliced 1 parsnip, sliced

1 red onion, sliced

Sea salt and ground black pepper, to taste 1 teaspoon paprika

Directions

Toss the beef roast with the mustard, apple juice, fish sauce, honey, dill and thyme in a glass bowl. Cover and let it marinate in your refrigerator overnight.

Add the marinated beef roast to the cooking basket, discarding the marinade.

Roast in your Air Fryer at 400 degrees F for 40 minutes. Turn the beef over and baste with the reserved marinade.

Add the carrots, parsnip and onion to the cooking basket; continue to cook for 12 minutes more. Season the beef and vegetables with salt, black pepper and paprika. Serve warm.

Greek-Style Roast Beef

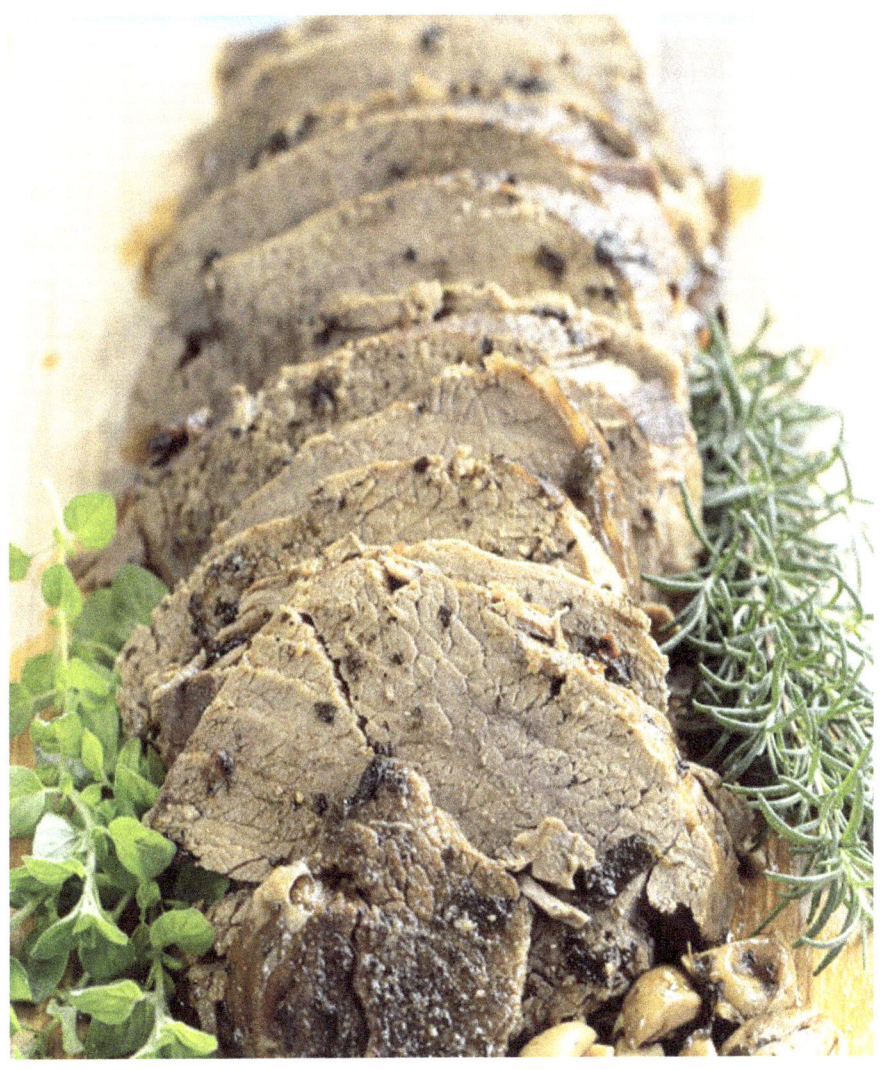

(Ready in about 55 minutes | Servings 3)

Per serving:

348 Calories; 16.1g Fat; 1.6g Carbs; 49g Protein; 0.9g Sugars

Ingredients

1 clove garlic, halved

1 ½ pounds beef eye round roast 1 zucchini, sliced lengthwise

2 teaspoons olive oil

1 teaspoon Greek spice mix Sea salt, to season

1/2 cup Greek-style yogurt

Directions

Rub the beef eye round roast with garlic halves.

Brush the beef eye round roast and zucchini with olive oil. Sprinkle with spices and place the beef in the cooking basket.

Roast in your Air Fryer at 400 degrees F for 40 minutes. Turn the beef over.

Add the zucchini to the cooking basket and continue to cook for 12 minutes more or until cooked through. Serve warm, garnished with Greek-style yogurt. Enjoy!

Italian Piadina Sandwich

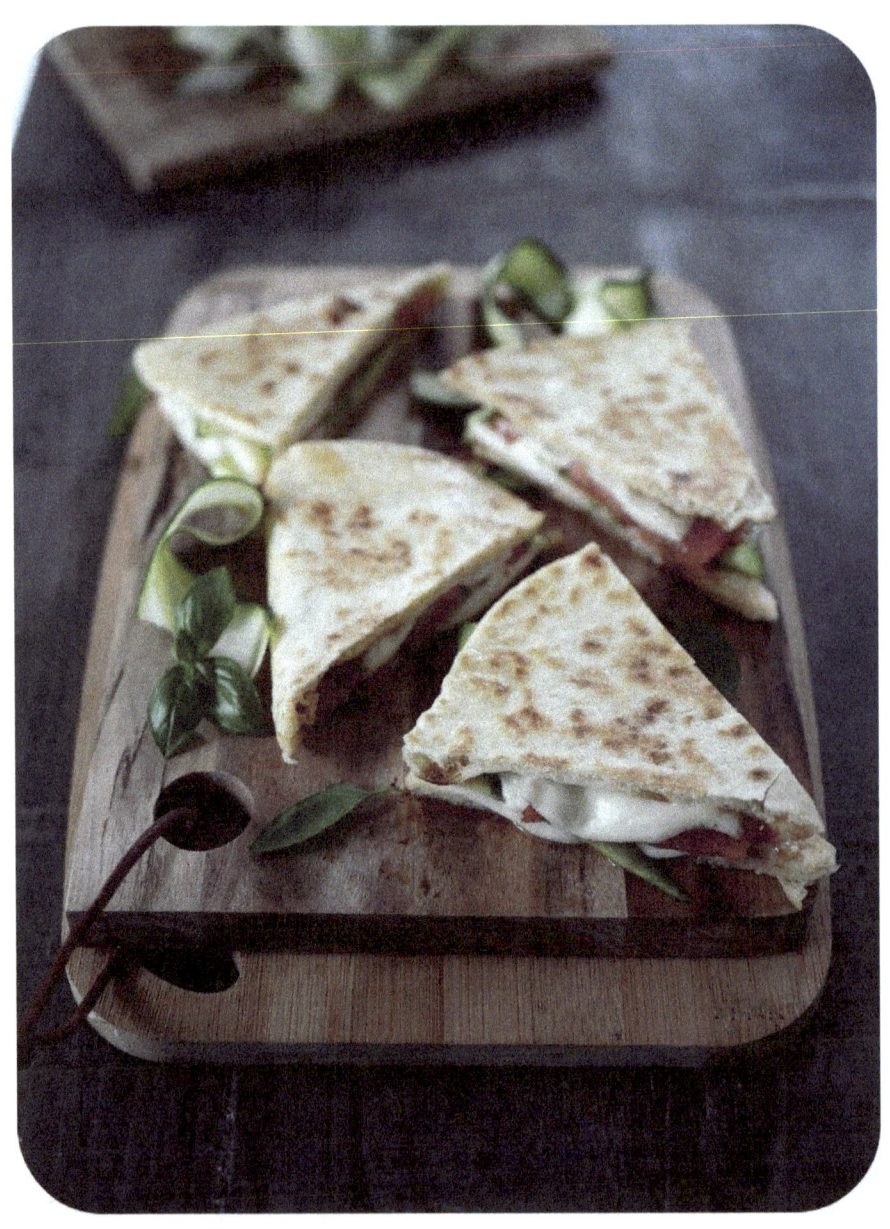

(Ready in about 20 minutes | Servings 2)

Per serving:

384 Calories; 24.8g Fat; 11.1g Carbs; 31.1g Protein; 4.9g Sugars

Ingredients

1/2 pound ribeye steak

1 teaspoon sesame oil

Sea salt and red pepper, to taste

2 medium-sized piadinas

2 ounces Fontina cheese, grated 4 tablespoons Giardiniera

Directions

Brush the ribeye steak with sesame oil and season with salt and red pepper.

Cook at 400 degrees F for 6 minutes. Then, turn the steak halfway through the cooking time and continue to cook for a further 6 minutes.

Slice the ribeye steak into bite-sized strips. Top the piadinas with steak strips and cheese.

Heat the sandwich in your Air Fryer at 380 degrees F for about 3 minutes until the cheese melts. Top with Giardiniera and serve.

Bon appétit!

Italian-Style Steak with Cremini Mushrooms

(Ready in about 15 minutes | Servings 2)

Per serving:

260 Calories; 12.4g Fat; 7.9g Carbs; 28.4g Protein; 4.7g Sugars

Ingredients

1/2 pound flank steak, cut into bite-sized pieces 8 ounces Cremini mushrooms, sliced

2 tablespoons tamari sauce

1 tablespoon peanut oil

1 teaspoon Italian seasoning blend Salt and black pepper, to taste

Directions

Toss the steak and mushrooms with tamari sauce, peanut oil, Italian spices, salt and black pepper. Toss until the steak and mushrooms are well coated on all sides.

Transfer the beef to the Air Fryer cooking basket. Cook at 400 degrees F for 7 minutes.

Then, shake the basket and stir in the mushrooms. Continue to cook for 5 minutes longer. Serve immediately.

London Broil with Herb Butter

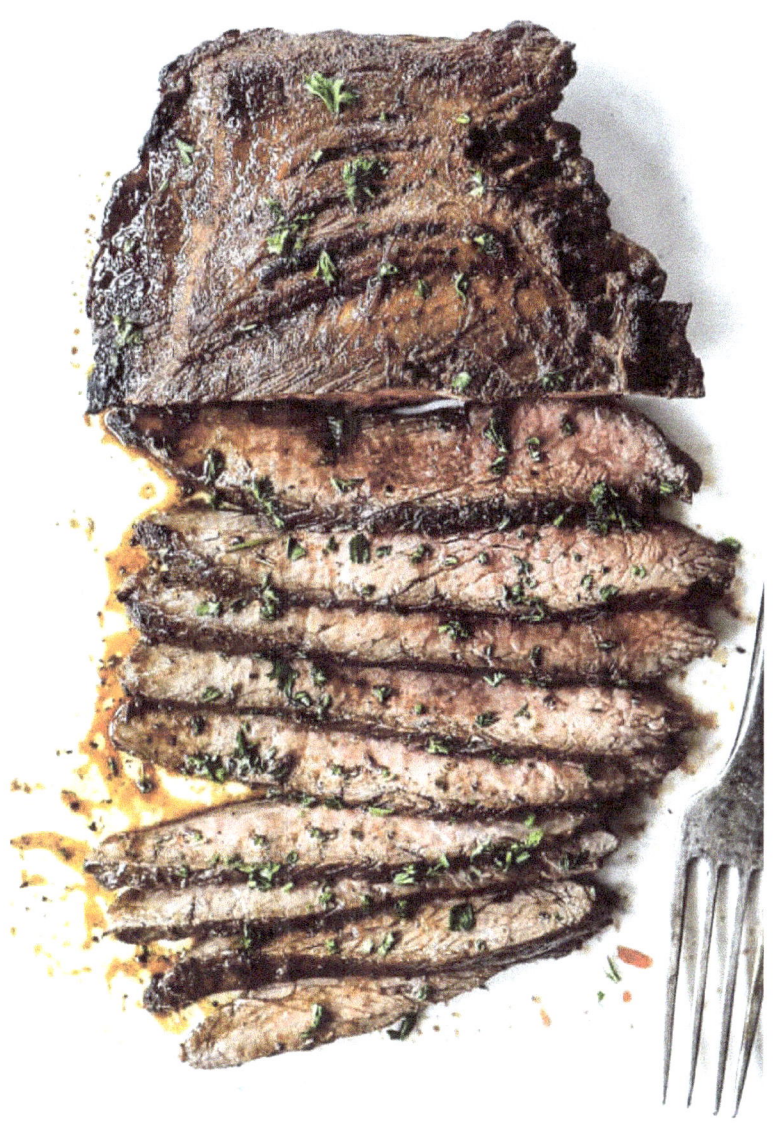

(Ready in about 30 minutes | Servings 3)

Per serving:

378 Calories; 21.3g Fat; 0.4g Carbs; 47g Protein; 0.3g Sugars

Ingredients

1 pound London broil Herb butter:

2 tablespoons butter, at room temperature

1 teaspoon basil, chopped

1 tablespoon cilantro, chopped 1 tablespoon chives, chopped 1 tablespoon lemon juice

Coarse sea salt and crushed black peppercorns, to taste

Directions

Pat the London broil dry with paper towels. Mix all Ingredients for the herb butter.

Cook in the preheated Air Fryer at 400 degrees F for 14 minutes; turn over, brush with the herb butter and continue to cook for a further 12 minutes.

Slice the London broil against the grain and serve warm.

Marinated London Broil

(Ready in about 25 minutes+ marinating time | Servings 2)

Per serving:

448 Calories; 22.6g Fat; 13.8g Carbs; 48g Protein; 11.7g Sugars

Ingredients

2 tablespoons soy sauce 2 garlic cloves, minced 1 teaspoon mustard

1 tablespoon olive oil

2 tablespoons wine vinegar 1 tablespoon honey

1 pound London broil 1/2 teaspoon paprika

Salt and black pepper, to taste

Directions

In a ceramic dish, mix the soy sauce, garlic, mustard, oil, wine vinegar and honey. Add in the London broil and let it marinate for 2 hours in your refrigerator.

Season the London broil with paprika, salt and pepper.

Cook in the preheated Air Fryer at 400 degrees F for 10 minutes; turn over and continue to cook for a further 10 minutes.

Slice the London broil against the grain and eat warm. Enjoy!

Mayo Roasted Sirloin Steak

(Ready in about 20 minutes | Servings 3)

Per serving:

418 Calories; 31.3g Fat; 0.2g Carbs; 30.1g Protein; 0.2g Sugars

Ingredients

1 pound sirloin steak, cubed 1/2 cup mayonnaise

1 tablespoon red wine vinegar 1/2 teaspoon dried basil

1 teaspoon garlic, minced

1/2 teaspoon cayenne pepper

Kosher salt and ground black pepper, to season

Directions

Pat dry the sirloin steak with paper towels.

In a small mixing dish, thoroughly combine the remaining Ingredients until everything is well incorporated.

Toss the cubed steak with the mayonnaise mixture and transfer to the Air Fryer cooking basket.

Cook in the preheated Air Fryer at 400 degrees F for 7 minutes. Shake the basket and continue to cook for a further 7 minutes. Bon appétit!

Meatballs with Cranberry Sauce

(Ready in about 40 minutes | Servings 4)

Per serving:

520 Calories; 22.4g Fat; 44g Carbs; 45.4g Protein; 25.5g Sugars

Ingredients

Meatballs:

1 ½ pounds ground chuck 1 egg

1 cup rolled oats

1/2 cup Romano cheese, grated 1/2 teaspoon dried basil

1/2 teaspoon dried oregano 1 teaspoon paprika

2 garlic cloves, minced

2 tablespoons scallions, chopped

Sea salt and cracked black pepper, to taste Cranberry Sauce:

10 ounces BBQ sauce

8 ounces cranberry sauce

Directions

In a large bowl, mix all Ingredients for the meatballs. Mix until everything is well incorporated; then, shape the meat mixture into 2-inch balls using a cookie scoop.

Transfer them to the lightly greased cooking basket and cook at 380 degrees F for 10 minutes. Shake the basket occasionally and work in batches.

Add the BBQ sauce and cranberry sauce to a saucepan and cook over moderate heat until you achieve a glaze-like consistency; it will take about 15 minutes.

Gently stir in the air fried meatballs and cook an additional 3 minutes or until heated through. Enjoy!

Mediterranean Burgers with Onion Jam

(Ready in about 20 minutes | Servings 2)

Per serving:

474 Calories; 26.5g Fat; 32.9g Carbs; 29g Protein; 26.1g Sugars

Ingredients

1/2 pound ground chuck

2 tablespoons scallions, chopped 1/2 teaspoon garlic, minced

1 teaspoon brown mustard

Kosher salt and ground black pepper, to taste 2 burger buns

2 ounces Haloumi cheese 1 medium tomato, sliced 2 Romaine lettuce leaves Onion jam:

2 tablespoons butter, at room temperature 2 red onions, sliced

Sea salt and ground black pepper, to taste 1 cup red wine

2 tablespoons honey

1 tablespoon fresh lemon juice

Directions

Mix the ground chuck, scallions, garlic, mustard, salt and black pepper until well combined; shape the mixture into two equal patties.

Spritz a cooking basket with a nonstick cooking spray. Air fry your burgers at 370 degrees F for about 11 minutes or to your desired degree of doneness.

Meanwhile, make the onion jam. In a small saucepan, melt the butter; once hot, cook the onions for about 4 minutes. Turn the heat to simmer, add salt, black pepper and wine and cook until liquid evaporates.

Stir in the honey and continue to simmer until the onions are a jam-like consistency; afterwards, drizzle with freshly squeezed lemon juice.

Top the bottom halves of the burger buns with the warm beef patty. Top with haloumi cheese, tomato, lettuce and onion jam.

Set the bun tops in place and serve right now. Enjoy!

Mediterranean-Style Beef Steak and Zucchini

(Ready in about 20 minutes | Servings 4)

Per serving:

396 Calories; 20.4g Fat; 3.5g Carbs; 47.8g Protein; 0.1g Sugars

Ingredients

1 ½ pounds beef steak 1 pound zucchini

1 teaspoon dried rosemary

1 teaspoon dried basil

1 teaspoon dried oregano

2 tablespoons extra-virgin olive oil 2 tablespoons fresh chives, chopped

Directions

Start by preheating your Air Fryer to 400 degrees F.

Toss the steak and zucchini with the spices and olive oil. Transfer to the cooking basket and cook for 6 minutes.

Now, shale the basket and cook another 6 minutes. Serve immediately garnished with fresh chives. Enjoy!

New York Strip with Mustard Butter

(Ready in about 20 minutes | Servings 4)

Per serving:

459 Calories; 27.4g Fat; 2.5g Carbs; 48.3g Protein; 1.4g Sugars

Ingredients

1 tablespoon peanut oil

2 pounds New York Strip 1 teaspoon cayenne pepper

Sea salt and freshly cracked black pepper, to taste 1/2 stick butter, softened

1 teaspoon whole-grain mustard

1/2 teaspoon honey

Directions

Rub the peanut oil all over the steak; season with cayenne pepper, salt, and black pepper.

Cook in the preheated Air Fryer at 400 degrees F for 7 minutes; turn over and cook an additional 7 minutes.

Meanwhile, prepare the mustard butter by whisking the butter, whole-grain mustard, and honey.

Serve the roasted New York Strip dolloped with the mustard butter. Bon appétit!

Peperonata with Beef Sausage

(Ready in about 35 minutes | Servings 4)

Per serving:

563 Calories; 41.5g Fat; 10.6g Carbs; 35.6g Protein; 7.9g Sugars

Ingredients

2 teaspoons canola oil 2 bell peppers, sliced

1 green bell pepper, sliced

1 serrano pepper, sliced 1 shallot, sliced

Sea salt and pepper, to taste

1/2 dried thyme

1 teaspoon dried rosemary 1/2 teaspoon mustard seeds 1 teaspoon fennel seeds

2 pounds thin beef parboiled sausage

Directions

Brush the sides and bottom of the cooking basket with 1 teaspoon of canola oil. Add the peppers and shallot to the cooking basket.

Toss them with the spices and cook at 390 degrees F for 15 minutes, shaking the basket occasionally. Reserve.

Turn the temperature to 380 degrees F

Then, add the remaining 1 teaspoon of oil. Once hot, add the sausage and cook in the preheated Air Frye for 15 minutes, flipping them halfway through the cooking time.

Serve with reserved pepper mixture. Bon appétit!

Porterhouse Steak with Tangy Sauce

(Ready in about 20 minutes | Servings 2)

Per serving:

309 Calories; 8.1g Fat; 12.3g Carbs; 42.5g Protein; 10.3g Sugars

Ingredients

1/2 pound Porterhouse steak, cut into four thin pieces Salt and pepper, to season

1 teaspoon sesame oil

1 teaspoon garlic paste 1 teaspoon ginger juice 1 tablespoon fish sauce 1 tablespoon soy sauce

1 habanero pepper, minced 2 tablespoons brown sugar

Directions

Pat the steak dry and generously season it with salt and black pepper.

Cook in the preheated Air Fryer at 400 degrees F for 7 minutes; turn on the other side and cook an additional 7 to 8 minutes.

To make the sauce, heat the remaining Ingredients in a small saucepan over medium-high heat; let it simmer for a few minutes until heated through.

Spoon the sauce over the steak and serve over hot cooked rice or egg noodles. Bon appétit!

Roasted Ribeye with Garlic Mayo

(Ready in about 20 minutes | Servings 3)

Per serving:

437 Calories; 24.8g Fat; 1.8g Carbs; 51g Protein; 0.1g Sugars

Ingredients

1 ½ pounds ribeye, bone-in

1 tablespoon butter, room temperature Salt, to taste

1/2 teaspoon crushed black pepper 1/2 teaspoon dried dill

1/2 teaspoon cayenne pepper

1/2 teaspoon garlic powder 1/2 teaspoon onion powder 1 teaspoon ground coriander 3 tablespoons mayonnaise

1 teaspoon garlic, minced

Directions

Start by preheating your Air Fryer to 400 degrees F.

Pat dry the ribeye and rub it with softened butter on all sides. Sprinkle with seasonings and transfer to the cooking basket.

Cook in the preheated Air Fryer for 15 minutes, flipping them halfway through the cooking time.

In the meantime, simply mix the mayonnaise with garlic and place in the refrigerator until ready to serve. Bon appétit!

Scotch Fillet with Sweet 'n' Sticky Sauce

(Ready in about 40 minutes | Servings 4)

Per serving:

556 Calories; 17.9g Fat; 25.8g Carbs; 60g Protein; 10.4g Sugars

Ingredients

2 pounds scotch fillet, sliced into strips 4 tablespoons tortilla chips, crushed

2 green onions, chopped

Sauce:

1 tablespoon butter

2 garlic cloves, minced

1/2 teaspoon dried rosemary 1/2 teaspoon dried dill

1/2 cup beef broth

1 tablespoons fish sauce 2 tablespoons honey

Directions

Start by preheating your Air Fryer to 390 degrees F.

Coat the beef strips with the crushed tortilla chips on all sides. Spritz with cooking spray on all sides and transfer them to the cooking basket.

Cook for 30 minutes, shaking the basket every 10 minutes.

Meanwhile, heat the sauce ingredient in a saucepan over medium-high heat. Bring to a boil and reduce the heat; cook until the sauce has thickened slightly.

Add the steak to the sauce; let it sit approximately 8 minutes. Serve over the hot egg noodles if desired.

Sunday Beef Schnitzel

(Ready in about 15 minutes | Servings 2)

Per serving:

501 Calories; 20.1g Fat; 24.1g Carbs; 54.3g Protein; 2g Sugars

Ingredients

2 beef schnitzel

Salt and black pepper, to taste 2 ounces all-purpose flour

1 egg, beaten

1/2 cup breadcrumbs 1/2 teaspoon paprika 1 teaspoon olive oil

1/2 lemon, cut into wedges to serve

Directions

Pat the beef dry and generously season it with salt and black pepper.

Add the flour to a rimmed plate. Place the egg in a shallow bowl and mix the breadcrumbs and paprika in another bowl.

Dip the meat in the flour first, then the egg, then the paprika/breadcrumb mixture. Drizzle olive oil over each beef schnitzel.

Cook in the preheated Air Fryer at 390 degrees F for about 10 minutes, flipping the meat halfway through the cooking time. Bon appétit!

Taco Stuffed Avocados

(Ready in about 15 minutes | Servings 3)

Per serving:

521 Calories; 42.1g Fat; 23.1g Carbs; 20.2g Protein; 4.8g Sugars

Ingredients

1/3 pound ground beef

2 tablespoons shallots, minced 1/2 teaspoon garlic, minced

1 tomato, chopped

1/3 teaspoon Mexican oregano Salt and black pepper, to taste

1 chipotle pepper in adobo sauce, minced 1/4 cup cilantro

3 avocados, cut into halves and pitted

1/2 cup Cotija cheese, grated

Directions

Preheat a nonstick skillet over medium-high heat. Cook the ground beef and shallot for about 4 minutes.

Stir in the garlic and tomato and continue to sauté for a minute or so. Add in the Mexican oregano, salt, black pepper, chipotle pepper and cilantro.

Then, remove a bit of the pulp from each avocado half and fill them with the taco mixture.

Cook in the preheated Air Fryer at 400 degrees F for 5 minutes. Top with Cotija cheese and continue to cook for 4 minutes more or until cheese is bubbly. Enjoy!

Tex-Mex Taco Pizza

(Ready in about 20 minutes | Servings 1)

Per serving:

686 Calories; 27.1g Fat; 72.4g Carbs; 40.2g Protein; 21.4g Sugars

Ingredients

1 teaspoon lard, melted

4 ounces ground beef sirloin 4 ounces pizza dough

2 tablespoons jarred salsa

1/4 teaspoon Mexican oregano 1/2 teaspoon basil

1/2 teaspoon granulated garlic 2 ounces cheddar cheese grated 1 plum tomato, sliced

Directions

Melt the lard in a skillet over medium-high heat; once hot, cook the beef until no longer pink, about 5 minutes.

Roll the dough out and transfer it to the Air Fryer cooking basket. Spread the jarred salsa over the dough.

Sprinkle Mexican oregano, basil, garlic and cheese over the salsa. Top with the sautéed beef, then with the sliced tomato.

Bake in your Air Fryer at 375 degrees F for about 11 minutes until the bottom of crust is lightly browned. Bon appétit!

Traditional Italian Beef Braciole

(Ready in about 15 minutes | Servings 4)

Per serving:

243 Calories; 13.1g Fat; 3.1g Carbs; 27g Protein; 1.6g Sugars

Ingredients

1 pound round steak, pounded 1/4 inch thick Sea salt and ground black pepper, to taste

1 tablespoon olive oil

1 red onion, sliced

1/4 cup provolone cheese, shredded 2 tablespoons marinara sauce

1 tablespoon fresh cilantro, chopped

1 tablespoon fresh Italian parsley, chopped 1 large Italian pepper, deveined and sliced

Directions

Pat the round steak dry with paper towels and generously season it with salt and black pepper.

Heat the olive oil in a small skillet over a moderate heat; once hot, sauté the onion until just tender and translucent.

Add in the cheese, marinara, cilantro, parsley and pepper; stir to combine well. Spoon the mixture onto the center of the steak.

Roll the steak jelly-roll style and secure with toothpicks.

Cook your Braciole in the preheated Air Fryer at 400 degrees F for about 10 minutes, checking the meat halfway through the cooking time.

Serve with hot cooked orecchiette pasta or polenta. Bon appétit!

Alphabetical Index

A

American-Style Roast Beef 1
Alphabetical Index 104
Argentinian Beef Empanadas 4
Authentic Greek Souvlaki with Sauce 7

B

Barbecue Skirt Steak 10
BBQ Glazed Beef Riblets 13
Beef and Broccoli Stir-Fry 16
Beef Parmigiana Sliders 19
Beef Sausage-Stuffed Zucchini 22
Beef Taco Roll-Ups with Cotija Cheese 25

C

Chicago-Style Beef Sandwich 28
Chuck Roast with Rustic Potatoes 31
Classic Beef Jerky 34
Crustless Beef and Cheese Tart 37
Cuban Mojo Beef 40

D

Dad's Barbecued Ribs 43
Dad's Meatloaf with a Twist 46
Dijon Top Chuck with Herbs 49
Doubly Cheesy Meatballs 51

E

Easy Beef Burritos 54

F

Filet Mignon and Green Bean Salad 57

G

Grandma's Meat Tarts 60
Grandma's Roast Beef with Harvest Vegetables 62
Greek-Style Roast Beef 65

I

Italian Piadina Sandwich 68
Italian-Style Steak with Cremini Mushrooms 71

L

London Broil with Herb Butter 73

M

Marinated London Broil 76
Mayo Roasted Sirloin Steak 78
Meatballs with Cranberry Sauce 80
Mediterranean Burgers with Onion Jam 82
Mediterranean-Style Beef Steak and Zucchini 84

N

New York Strip with Mustard Butter 86

P

Peperonata with Beef Sausage 88
Porterhouse Steak with Tangy Sauce 90

R

Roasted Ribeye with Garlic Mayo 92

S

Scotch Fillet with Sweet 'n' Sticky Sauce 94
Sunday Beef Schnitzel 96

T

Taco Stuffed Avocados 98
Tex-Mex Taco Pizza 100

Traditional Italian Beef Braciole 102

www.ingramcontent.com/pod-product-compliance
Lightning Source LLC
Chambersburg PA
CBHW071008080526
44587CB00015B/2383